PREFACE

The reason and whole purpose of this book is to help educate the fight world, as well as the world in general about what 52 Blocks is. Some may not need an introduction, but others may. Carolina Chaos is a style of 52 Blocks founded and developed by me. Its telling people about the diversity and the different methods of 52 Blocks that is taught throughout the world. This book has its urgency when it comes to the education of 52 Blocks and its culture. Reasons on why it was developed and reasons for which it may be altered for the advantage of the practitioner.

This book came about when I decided that 52 Blocks was a style that needed to be expanded to the world, primarily the fight world. It has been show cased in movies and documentaries, but never in dept and with explanations on its techniques, why and how we use it. I chose to write this book because of the love of the art, and the compassion I have towards the martial arts in general. Brining to the world 52 Blocks Carolina Chaos is my brain child, and yours to read, understand, as well as possibly educate. Life in general has motivated me to put my thoughts and experiences on paper. Through my many years of competing professionally in Kickboxing, Karate, Boxing, and Mixed Martial Arts. I live to teach, and instruct those that wish to learn and excel in the art form of 52 Blocks as well anything they choose to pursue in life.

My inspirations are people that I highly respect. I have been in the martial arts for 34 yrs. And I credit instructors like John Orsmby, Bill McDonald, Dale Frye, my 52 Blocks Mentor and friend Daniel Marks out of Constellation 52 Global who has helped to elevate the art of 52 Blocks and has become a pioneer of this amazing art form. These men have not only been warriors of the martial art, but friends as well that gave me something that could not be bought. And that is trust, loyalty and friendship While writing this book, I have learned that my love for the art is not selfish, and through my experience's this information would allow someone else to take the journey of learning and instructing just as I did.

Carolina Chaos: 52 Blocks

From the begging of time there has been acts of war, and some form of conflict and numerous accounts of violence that has plagued our existence. So we are no strangers to an unsettling shift of uncomfortable living environments. Sometimes these acts could be avoided and sometimes they are encouraged through various choices that are being made purposely just to appease ones ego. But to each his own, and to each his own down fall.

What makes our life worth defending? What is our reason to defend? These are valid questions, and the way the world is today, preparation is key.

Are you prepared, are you aware of the Chaos that has engulf the world? Lets enter the world of 52 Blocks, Lets visit its style of Carolina Chaos.

Chaos: Disorder, Confusion, Disarray, Mayhem, HAVOC, and acts of Disruption.

Such a nasty word Chaos seems to be for too many people. But in the world of 52 Blocks it could be music to some practitioners ears. Many may know how to use it to their advantage, but it has to be understood to be effective. To be fair, we may have some newbie's to the lifestyle of 52 Blocks, so to give them the style of Carolina Chaos: 52 Blocks would be like giving a 2 month old baby a pound of steak for breakfast. So let me first introduce the original 52 Blocks and some of its information, history, names, and key components of this art that many people didn't know existed, and many martial artist didn't know was a real martial art that was reared and respected then, and now. It is still evolving, and students of the craft continues to grow throughout the world and it will not cease due to the ongoing popularity of celebrities and athletes that choose to explore 52 Blocks as a way of life.

Carolina: Of course North Carolina, South Carolina are states in which we have practitioners live, but its history to the name Carolina. Keeping it simple and to the point. There are historic stories dealing with where Carolina originated from, but in the case of 52 Block Carolina Chaos is different.

Historically Carolina means Freeman or Freeholder.

Breaking it down to a Free man without any bondage. Carolina Chaos puts a man with a style of fighting that creates a free Rhythm of Combat and that is fluid, loose and devastating. And a man with an Agenda to destroy you with his hands cannot be stopped, he will use all avenues to his advantage, all techniques and every ounce of energy to make sure you are subdued or takeout by any means necessary. Carolina Chaos is a consistent flow of movement with the feet, hands, head, shoulders and using angles to his advantage. Wild, but controlled. Controlled Chaos is the aspect of Carolina Chaos, and will give the 52 Blocker the advantage of surprise attacks, and sharp execution of techniques that will remain effective in a defensive situation, or when you feel the need to engage.

The art of 52 Blocks has said the have been forged in the prison system and mastered on the streets. That is true in some aspects, but others seem to be unclear about its true origins. 52 Pickup is how it got its name, derived from a card game, it stated let the cards fall where they may, also saying anything goes. Although what is true, is that it has been mastered on the streets of New York City and has spread abroad through the East Coast and slowly making its way to the Midwestern parts of the country. 52 Blocks is a deceptive martial art, and has become a dangerous style of fighting. Flashy and very tricky to the eye, but also very deadly and complex. With this, 52 Blocks is indeed different from all other styles of fighting. Boxing is the base style, but there are added techniques that help create 52 Blocks and separate its movements and skill level to a whole new horizon.

Some techniques of the art of 52 Blocks are named from different aspects of the streets, prison system, as well as professional fight organizations. But the only difference from 52 Blocks and the professional fight arena is that there are no rules or restrictions. You have different styles or methods of 52 Blocks, they all have territorial bias, while some practice a style from Harlem NY, you also have others adding to, or taking away techniques that may reign in Long Island, Staten Island, or the Bronx. So many different sets, and areas throughout New York City compete to see whose 52 Blocks techniques are the most effective. It's all for the practitioner. Some of the techniques of 52 Blocks which are practiced on the Eastern part of the country are and can be different, but still highly effective. It is still 52 Blocks, but executed in fashions that suit the person that is using the movements. Some are tight, some are flashy. Some are basic and to the point, nothing more nothing less. Again it is all based on the way it present yourself, and being able to asset the situation that you are in at that particular moment.

Carolina Chaos

&

Its Diversities

Taking nothing away from the 52 Blocks system, it thrives on its deceptiveness, its cunning and mobility. The use of additional hand movements give the 52 Hand blocks system its advantage. Carolina Chaos however depletes energy during movement so each technique is effective when thrown as a fake feint, or primary attack. There is never a difference in the blocking or attacking with the original 52 Blocks and Carolina Chaos style of fighting. But diversity or a proven enhanced method to deliver more precise techniques which in turn could help develop an impregnable defense that cannot be matched. Mike Tyson spoke of his attacks as being vicious, the same can be said about Carolina Chaos. It is a vicious style, it is actually a state of being in a Controlled Chaos mindset with defensive techniques as well as offensive. Again, taking nothing away from the original system, Carolina Chaos is compelled to bringing a diverse dimension to fighting which goes beyond the streets, but on another level of combat that could be used in an arena or combat sports environment. The technical execution of moments and skills are truly mind blowing to view, and difficult to understand if you are not trained in the art form of 52 Blocks fighting systems. Other martial artists or historians may think differently, but they can only speculate and try to reveal and weakness they see by sitting at a desk and reading documents, or viewing content on social media or the world wide web. But they are all entitled to their own opinions, at least until the step foot in the square, and let the cards fall where they may. Many will not agree to the statement, but there is only one way to prove a point, and that is to fight.

Now as we spoke briefly about diversity and similarities in the 52 Block systems.

In earlier texts we spoke about the various boroughs and sets. Practitioners throughout the country "perform" if you will, their renditions of 52 Hand blocks in ways that may look unfamiliar, or in some cases wrong. But there is no truth to that matter. Styles differ in the world of 52, blocks change, they are used differently, and are called different name. With this, these techniques are not wrong, just labeled and used according to ones skill set or demographic style. But to be clear, there is no set demographic aspect when it come to area of practicing 52 Blocks. But you do have East Coast, and the West Coast 52 blockers attempting to make their craft one in a million, but that is in a short word impossible. The Midwest may have applied a new skill set based on who the teacher is, and how their training has either masked or revealed there concepts to make it look different, but have the same effects. Now, with this, it doesn't make any part of the country better, it only unites the 52 Block community and allows us a brotherhood/ and or sisterhood to come together and make this art form one of the most credible and effective martial arts out there. It's all about style and the level of execution. It's how you flow with what you have, and whether or not you could make it effective against an attack being it's against another 52 Blocker or any style of fighting. The variations are key when in the arena of our art form, it's all in who executes. Execution is the Key, and with this you find yourself struggling with why techniques won't work, and why they are not in line with what you perceived in your mind when you began your thought process before the fight began. Never start what you cannot finish.

The Importance of Execution

It's not rocket science when they say execution of a technique is critical to the art of 52 blocks. Throwing punches, blocks and takedowns have to be done properly if you expect results, that is why we train. Apply what we learn, and get what we need done effectively offensively and defensively. If you are unsure of your technique, " Then Don't Throw it" Being aware of the specific technique are preparing to throw is very critical to the success of a fight. The only result that matters is survival and the victory. Although 52 Blocks has methods of which you **Pause and Stall and Bail** during attacks, you must also learn to pace them and create a balance with these methods in order to witness success of the particular movement. Practice consistency and be consistent when you practice, this creates perfection and allows you to correct mistakes and weakness that could sew up the holes in your game. Never be afraid to throw punches, elbows, knees, and trips when in combat, versatility is key in creating an offensive barrage, and a defensive game plan. They are all made to do damage, hurt and mame and disable your attacker/enemy. You have to position yourself to make contact and react accordingly. The importance of execution tells you in a nut shell that whenever you execute a strike you are out to hurt someone, you want to make contact consistently and you really want to do damage at a scale of 110.

There is only one way to train, one way to prepare and one way to secure victory, and that is through training of the body and mind. Sure is it clique but it's the for sure truth and there is no way around it.

Development & Conditioning

The development that comes with learning 52 Hand Blocks is not a simple task, but far from difficult . This is a style of fighting that you won't need any prior experience with fighting or training. The simplicity of the movements are manageable for small to large framed practitioners. Pictures and illustrations will be provided for visuals and examples. But with visual examples they mean nothing without putting in work with a physically target, training partners, and or opponents. Using Thai pads, hand mitts, and body shields are key to being accurate and sharp. Proper technique brings speed, speed brings power, power brings explosiveness. The developmental stages of 52 Blocks consists of proper movements, observing patterns and tendencies and adjusting to momentum. Developing is watching and watching is learning. Learning is again executing common sense.

More on development in later chapters of the text Chronicles of King Agrippa. Allow what is taken in be processed, so that the mind will stay sharp and the body a total weapon both mentally and physically. Patience will always be a virtue, but destruction should be second to that when it comes to the actual use of the style of 52 hand blocks. With any art, discipline , or style you have to condition yourself. Your mind as well as your body has to be conditioned in order to function properly. When I speak of the word function, I am talking about application and evaluation. In order to execute and execute properly, one must be conditioned and conditioned in the proper ways of the system of 52 Blocks. Each art has their own ways of prepare the body, a 52 Blockers condition themselves on a level of superhuman status.

Stamina, Endurance, Strength, Balance, Agility, and the Intestinal fortitude. This goes without saying that the physical man is important, but the mental game is the main focus and strength of the style. Physiologically you have to be on point, knowing how to work your opponents mind, screw with it to win the battle, and dismantle it when it's time for the return war. Sure it is a very it is a very physical style of fighting, and you will see grueling training involved in its development and conditioning process. The conditioning strengthen the heart and body hardening areas that will make you a force to deal with. It also gives the lower body its smooth flow needed to evade and out maneuver your opponent.

Agility is the key to movement within the 52 Blocks arena. Footwork drills, sprawls, burpees and other methods are very important when you are working with agility drills, they tend to keep you sharp and balanced when you are at completeness.

Strength training goes into the area of 52 Blocks by simply using a lot of body weight exercises. In order to be effective there must be some form of muscle exertion and that takes consistency, and some weight training, some stress on the other hand your discretion is yours and yours alone.

Carolina Chaos Style of 52 Blocks pushes minimal weight training and lots of Bodyweight exercise, pushups, sit-ups, free squats, pull ups, chin ups, burpees, mountain climbers, Kamikaze pushups, Knuckle pushups, etc. These are some core and advanced exercises that can be utilized to incorporate strength, speed, agility and stamina. Being lean and compact is not a necessity to the art of 52 Blocks. It is indeed a broken purpose. But larger practitioners have the advantage also, Such as strength, leverage and the defensive prowess.

Each body make up is key to one's own victory, or his or her own defeat. Focus on what is being done at that particular time. Always stress caution because we don't know who we are up against, and how much training they have done.

Jumping rope, sprinting up a steep hill, jumping jacks, long distance running at a slow and moderate pace, then full blast for about 20 seconds. Skipping while you run freely or on a treadmill if available. Striking focus mitts at a consistent and fast pace not really focusing on speed but technique and power. This creates muscle endurance and enables one to fight for a long period of time while still remaining effective and sharp. Being sloppy isn't a trait of a seasoned 52 blocker Carolina Chaos style practitioner. We remain sharp and always demonstrates a form of controlled chaos which could sometimes rival other methods in which 52 Blocks are executed. Make the opponent underestimate you and your craft. Repetition is the key to everything, but strategy also plays a part. You don't want to be handled or picked off because you are telegraphing your technique and using them in the same order and tell tale patterns. Meaning repeating the same sequence of techniques and movements where the opponent can capitalize and prevent you from coming at them with a full barrage of effective techniques. That would be the best example of complacency. You are the one that prevents the failure of being complacent. You are the one that creates the opportunity and prevent the hole and all other weakness that may occur when practicing, competing or just working movements. Again the experience will come as your level of learning increases. With this, your level of learning could consist of quite a few avenues. Visuals, hands on and text, bearing you are able to use all these factors consistently and openly with a partner. This all starts with proper training and conditioning. You cannot be an effective fighter if you don't put in the training and work first.

Block and Shield

Incorporation and balance makes the technique work for you. First, understand the execution of the technique that you are throwing, What it does, why it is executed, how to execute it, how to counter it, and if it can be countered. Proper utilization of this skill, and the ability to be mobile with its methods of movements, and tactics. Being defensive is the primary mission of the 52 Blocks system. The blocks are those to simply **Block and Shield** and used as a defensively as a weapon to again, defend one's self as well as a third party. Passive yet aggressive, 52 Block serves it purpose, and gets the job done no matter the conditions. Block and shield can be executed anyway that you like, as long as it serves it purpose on the offensive and or defensive side. There are ways to alter and make Block and Shield you own, but that truly comes from experience and repetition. Respect the art of 52 Blocks, don't allow yourself to create useless techniques, that will degrade and deem the art useless. There are phonies and copy cats out there that will claim the art form to be BS, but those are the ones that have not seen combat or given or taken a whooping. Strive to keep your craft sharp, and undeniably Chaotic. Take pride and don't disrespect the Craft Most importantly, don't even think about disrespecting yourself. It will only dishonor you as a person, and your technique and YOUR credentials. Being aware, and taking responsibility for what you learn, who you learn it from and how you present will say a lot to those that put in hours, days, nights, and years of training to bring 52 Blocks to the top tier of fighting, but it cannot be done with weak hearted wannabe fighters that don't respect the craft, or themselves. Don't let your instructor name be mud by using his name to promote your garbage technique. It happens all the time and pride is on the line.

Putting in the best foods

will result in a well oiled

Machine

When you put healthy substances in your body and protect it, you body will protect you. Premium gas in a car gives you premium performance, and poor gas gives you poor performance. It goes without saying, you are what you eat. And I believe that to be true.

Fruits, Veggies that are colorful and a wealth good for the body. Coconut oil, Peanut Oil are some great oils for the body.

Eating plenty of fish, preferably baked or grilled. Grilled Chicken, backed Chicken. Tuna, Salmon, White fish are great examples of good protein and brain food.

Grass fed beef, Bison are strong red meat sources of protein, try and get that in with your workouts and see a dynamic change in your body with strength and overall muscle gains.

Steamed Veggies, not over cooked

Calcium for strong bones

Amino Acids

Fish oil tablets for omega-3 heart health

Balanced diet

Try to avoid White rice, Breads, starches like pasta and potatoes, try and avoid these when possible. You never have to cut them out, but dropped them down to very low levels of consumption.

1 cheat day a week, pretty much anything you want. But only 1 day!

We are creating lean strong, healthy warriors and we strive to keep them balanced.

You want to try and drink at least 1 gallon of water a day.

No additives like juice packs or subs.

It's good to get green tea in your body, it provides energy and antioxidants and helps to flush out impurities.

Get a good multi-vitamin in your system at least a 3 month cycle. Drink plenty of water to balance the vitamin intake daily.

Incorporate Protein shakes an minimum of 3 times a week, and if you are preparing them for yourself to gain bulk, use whole milk. But if you are looking for the lean machine, use filtered water or skim milk.

A good deter once a month is good to cleanse the body and flush out impurities and unwanted bloating and fat. But again keep your water intake intact.

Get plenty of rest, at least strive for 7 to 8 hours. You must recuperate in order to heal, and be effective during training, and or in a fight. Sleep is a must and it clears you mind so that you may focus and give 100 percent in all you do throughout the day. Combining all these methods will help complete a great cycle of healthy living and practice of 52 Hand blocks. Nothing is ever set in stone when it comes to nutrition, but these methods and ideas were given solely based on my experience in the fight game and overall awareness of the body and the mind. The importance of hydration, proper nutrition and taking care of your body are key to a long life. These ideas, methods and suggestions are never a promise of eternal life. But it will make you feel you can live forever. If you look at how the Spartans did it back in the early days of true warrior combat, they did not eat anything but one meal a day. And it was a very large meal at that. They had to fight for their meals. After a victorious battle, they were rewarded with large amounts of food.

Deliverance from Evil

You have a variety of Martial Arts in the world. The vast majority are compiled of tons of offensive techniques and skill sets. But when measuring all of these arts, they are known as self defense systems point blank. And this is nothing different from the 52 Blocks Carolina Chaos style of fighting.

52 Blocks is a defensive style that incorporates offensive prowess. Defending one's self is the

primary purpose of 52 Blocks. During the time of defense there is offensive explosions, or in the world of 52 Blocks its known as "Controlled Chaos"

You have to control the radius around you with precision, grace and a mind of survival with the ability to learn from the situation, or adapt to it at least, and live to tell about it. With this, it initiates instruction, and with instruction comes repetition and mastery. You have to stand and deliver yourself from evil. Evil being a barrage of attacks from every corner in your square. A consistent machine that rotates consistently in a circle and at various angles. Evil comes in many different shapes and forms, it's up to you to train the body and prepare for attacks via through one or more attackers. You will have fists, kicks, knees, elbows and a lot of clinches. When it comes to combat, through repetition and consistent studying of the art you will find yourself adapting to the evils of the strikes and clinches by preparing for them in bulk and not as single strikes like haymakers or cheap shots. An open mind creates and avenue of strategic choice that could cause you to survival a fight regardless of the outcome and provide a plan to improve on the next threat that may arise. The importance of defense in any art of fighting will always be key to survival and knowledge. If you cannot defend yourself, they your offense is pointless, and the fight is lost or the time of instruction was a waste of time and energy. Practice does make perfect, but consistency of proper techniques, movements and the act of patience prevents unwarranted failure. Unwarranted failure cannot be tolerated in 52 Blocks, it is a life or death situation that you only have one shot at. Make it count or make arrangements for your burial, because it would be certain death based on mistakes that are made. With this being said, Deliverance for Evil is simply put and should be well documented and understood. We cannot progress with a simple mindset of the world is all good, because it's not. Evil is forever present, and you have to be ready for any act of evil or ill will that may occur at any occasion. Defend, attack, evaluate, and Evade, keep this in mind and you will find yourself alive to tell the story of survival and victory at the same time, and prepare yourself for the next battle if and when it ever occurs. Just think about it and use logic, Is it true to think the way I teach is real or walk around feeling that there is no threat to you?

Superb technique
creates remarkable offense

How many times you can hit a person may seem impressive to some people. But to others, not so much. Quality in most cases are far more important than quantity. This is thinking with a level head and a conditioned mind. Providing if you are a fighter or someone this is merely training. Volume sometimes could be the main focus when it comes to delivering damage or achieving an objective. But having the perfect technique could end a fight with that one blow verses 3 or 4 sloppy techniques that could prolong an unwanted, and dangerous situation.

You look at legends like "Mother Dear" in Rijkers Island State Prison in NY, he was a convict with the sickest form of 52 Blocks. Famous and unstoppable until his demise by rival gang members within the system. They took him out with multiple attackers, being nobody could beat him one on one, or two on one, not even three on one. But nothing is fair in the prison system. There are many stories that float around saying he was killed many different ways and by different gang affiliates. But nobody truly knows the truth. But the bottom line is that he did live and he died one of the baddest dudes to every master 52 Blocks. Being who Mother Dear was, life behind the wall you could say was golden. He was the man on the yard, he was feared and respected when it came to having an outstanding knuckle game an no fear of what could happen on the yard. His technique was superb, that was because he practiced his craft consistently, from what is understood, he had no flaws in his game. Despite his death/murder coming through organized gang activity, AKA being jumped by multiple attackers with shanks and bangers. It showed that it takes more than one to take out a "Skilled" 52 Blocker.

But the point is if your offense is more than ready, your defense will shine because of the fact you cannot be hit. With this, you will be too busy throwing hands and elbows that they won't have time to throw anything back at you effectively. It's all about being active, being consistent and providing that massive offensive barrage that will blind and incapacitate your opponent. You also have to realize that when you find yourself busy and active you will always be ahead of the fight, and winning before he even realizes the fight has started. Take light into all situations, be ready so you won't have to get ready.

52 Blocks, when you hear this you ask are there only 52 Blocks in the system? No it was just a name given,

and derived from the 52 pickup card game. But to be honest it is hard to say because you have so many different practitioners making up techniques that may be a part of their style or to only make an extension of one technique that creates 2 separate blocks off of one side or one hand. They could be multiple blocks, so you could say it's more than 52 individual blocks. But too many is never a problem as long as it serves its purpose. Keep in mind 52 Blocks came from a card game which means "Let the cards fall where they may" or anything goes. No rules, no restrictions and limitless offensive techniques which in turns brings about Carolina Chaos, a method of continuous movements and strategies that only allow you to bring forth pain, confusion and making your opponent vulnerable and subject to consistent attacks. So be sure to build and perfect your craft with limitless offense and with that your techniques need to be superb. Make it happen by being under proven fighters with professional experience and or a true street fighting game that has been witnessed and tested on more than one occasion. Then and only then will you know what is viable and facts within the persons fight game and overall ability.

Know your techniques and there purposes. Understand what the jab does how it is thrown and why its thrown and more importantly when to throw it. It's useless and dumb to want to throw something you know nothing about only because you seen somebody else throw it on TV, or in some random fight. Prove the technique works before using on the street. That is what sparring and training with partners are for. Put in work to so that nobody would put that work on you. Practice the punch, or technique on a heavy bag, focus mitts, or again a live sparring partner that has some experience. You will never learn by sparring scrubs or guys that are not on your level. But then again you can always learn something from anyone, your game could never be so tight that you cannot seek correction, someone could see something you cannot, and when they correct you, it's your responsibility to learn from it and move forward by giving credit where credit its due. Once this is done, you can now add it to your arsenal of skills.

 Be sure to show and prove. That is the only way to gain respect and notoriety with the craft and your name. Take is seriously and make your name your BRAND. Your brand provides a lifetime of power within yourself. And this starts with your inner self, it begins with confidence in what you are learning and being able to take control over your mind and let it control your body. Your body doesn't tell you what to do, it's your mind, that is the strongest tool when it comes to learning, instructing and fighting. You can change it, make it better and allow it to grow and mature. You know yourself and it's up to you to again build yourself and extend your own legacy.

What people fail to realize is in training, what doesn't kill you makes you 10 times stronger. Surround yourself with people who have the same drive and determination as you do. There is strength in numbers and strength comes with unity in training an sharing ideas, concepts and training failures. There isn't any true division in the world of 52 Blocks, you do have various sets, and different groups that represent one particular instructor or region though out the country. But we all represent the same movement of 52 Blocks. There is no wrong way to present the art of 52 hand blocks because you have had so many people train in it from the early 70's, 80's and 90's. But there is this thing that we call "Evolution". It happens and in some instances it improves what is not broken, or enhances a proven style or art form, and there is nothing wrong with positive change, even if it's not broken. Some may disagree with what they see, and they have that right. But if its proven, then you find yourself questioning yourself based on the old ways and the new ways. Being effective is the whole point, and the only point that really matters.

But in defense to that notion, nobody wants to show and prove, they only talk and try to pimp the art form and recreate the movements and methods.

So that is when the REAL 52 Blockers come in to play and correct the frauds. Some new school practitioners need lessons on respect and honor, but that is only to be done and said properly and in an organized manner. We are not a gang to go and act as hooligans, we are a movement that present ourselves as warriors of 52 Blocks, we are still striving to get our respect in the world of Martial Arts, and going in head first like thugs is not the way to do it. Respect for the art needs to be re-established and a standard needs to be set and kept in the accordance to how 52 Hand Blocks should be practiced, and that is properly and consistently based on how it was taught in the old school. How they fought in prison, and on the streets, how it was meant to be used, and that was as a way of self expression, and way of self-defense, and more importantly a way of life. Why do you use 52 Blocks?

Is it for the love of the movement, or for show. Be wisely because you have some that live this life, and are proud of being called a 52 Blocker.

Combinations, Offense, Defense And the Powers Thereof

Everyone claims to have a fight game. Well most that say that they are fighters and really not.

You can dream of a superior arsenal of techniques and movements that could put your opponent on the ground and wow all the spectators witnessing the skills you produced to keep him down.. Now, with that being said, you have fighters out there that may have an awesome array of skills, and or combinations. Then you have those that have that One Hitter Quitter, now that is no real technique, but it has proven itself in world of fighting. One shot given, one body hit's the ground. This is when a man or woman can take a punch and hit someone with it and the fight is abruptly ended.. There is nothing wrong with that, but it can't work for everyone. But today's fighter are warriors now, they train to be ready so they won't have to get ready when it it's time to throw down, or defend one's self or a third party. Combinations are a sure fire way to improve your chances of winning a fight and surviving a hard fought battle. Use the many tools that you may have to complete your objective, and that is objective is to win.

What are you techniques? Do you know them and can you apply them when needed? As I said before in earlier text, Know your Craft.

 You have to look at basic punches and you have to analyze them. There based off the old sweet science of boxing. Boxing seem to be the primary base to a lot of martial arts style. Jabs, uppercuts, crosses are key to a good solid style of fighting, a good base. What is your base for your style? Think about it and you will see that boxing is in it and is hard to remove even if you wanted to.

- Jab
- Straight punch/Cross
- Hook
- Uppercut

These are some of your base punch that we use in the art of 52 Blocks. They are basic punches use to set of advance techniques and movements. When it pertains to boxing, kickboxing, and other striking arts, this is what you will see in its base.

These techniques are plain and simple to most boxers and or strikers. But 52 Blocks they learn how to alter these techniques and use them for the benefit of the objective. There are Smart, Sharp, and Clever uses for each technique. Throwing punches from the hip, from your knees and from any angle that may seem cumbersome or unusual to other fighters, will be your primary strength. But know that they are balanced and strategically thought out before even attempting to execute the one technique or skill sets. Examples are many, but once understood then and only then will you be able to execute them on your own.

Here are a few combinations and skills that are key to the art of 52 Blocks Carolina Chaos. The names of skills and techniques will be explained in detailed later in the text.

- 1, 2, Tyson (2x) clinch, Head Job, Shoulder Push, Pivot out at angle.
- 1,2,3, Take it Back, Rob the Bank (2x) Straight Blast Pivot (2x) out at angle.
- 1,2 to mid section Close Door (2x) Hand Rolls, 1 Hand of God, Pivot out at angle.

- 1,1 Sparta, Pivot out at angle, Maze Runner into Kryptonite, Pivot out with Peek-a-Boo end with Skull and Crossbones
- Peek-a-Boo (2x) 1,2,3, Devil's Elbow, 2 Spinning back fist, Inside leg kick, Hand of God, Shoulder Push Pivot out at angle.
- 1,2 Clinch, Complete Silence, Head Job, Busting Rocks, Make 'em Limp, Shoulder Push, transition to take down, Pivot out.

These combination sets are example of striking and moving in bulk. Staying fluid and active at all times is key to providing your opponent with true 52 Blocks experience. A total mixture of techniques and skill sets, blocks and movements, strategies as well. They may seem confusing, but they are actually very effective if practiced on a consistent basis and the proper format taught by a 52 blocks instructor.

Shutter Down	Remove the Crown
Close the door	Charlie's Horse
Skull and Crossbones	Devils Elbow

Take it Back	Hand of God
Rob the Bank	Broken Arrow

These are some of the blocks and attacks used in 52 Blocks Carolina Chaos style of fighting. Each have their own meaning and uses for various technique thrown from any angle.

The names are different, and were given for a purpose of its own. Each one of these are used to attack and block different technique skill sets. Though none are made to be 100 % full proof, but it's up to you the practitioner to execute show and prove and use them to provide the defense needed for survival. When you get in your mind to become great at something, you will be. Make sure you devote real time to what you want, then go and get it. Don't wait till it's too late. Apply the will to do what you are destined to do, and that is to become a fighting machine. You should your style, you make the move and you absorb the energy that is given free to those who wants to learn. That is a true warrior, and you will find yourself in a world of positive energy that makes you who you are and that is a fighter.

Strategic Movements

(No)body fights standing still, or keeps themselves dormant in one place while in battle. You have to be mobile and when you move you have to be strategic while doing it.

When you move, you must move with a purpose. Maneuver as if you are guiding missiles into orbit, or merely playing chess with and accomplished Grandmaster. Don't just move because you can, move because you have to. Make space, use angles and surprise opponents by constant movement and fluidity. You think when the Military get orders to go into battle, they grab their guns and gear and go. No that is not the case. They have to plan, and plan well. Strategic Movements are required for a reason, and that is to secure victory, and assure that all of the soldiers are safe. That is the same for fighting, you have to have Strategic Movements

Body Trickery

A lot of people follow their eyes when in a fight, they don't focus on the movements of a person, but on the movements of shoulders, arms, and torso. Now with Body Trickery, the rolling with the hands and shoulder brushes. There is a variety of faints and parries that would be appropriate with any technique, and its really up to how you want to display your skills and when you want to allow your opponent to witness them. As my Mentor has shared with me, moving your body to a rhythm, like a dance is what 52 Blocks is all about. With this, you are able to move your body and throw techniques from any angle simply because your body is moving as a fluid unit. There is not room for wasted movements, so make all of them count. Because a lot of times in a full blown fight, you only get once chance to get the win, if not, they will have the opportunity to knock you head off. Your choice.

There are techniques that we call detractor that could be used to set up different types of techniques.

Detractors are attention getters, or ground shakers. They are meant to fool, trick, and confuse your opponent while fighting or training. They could be used to set up and provide leverage to strategically end a fight that was initially never meant to be started. Detractors activate nerves, cause pain and gives you the advantage when you are trying to diminish the opponents confidence. You choose the way to activate a detractor, they could save your life in different situations. And it would make you have a level of confidence that can give your game a sharpness and look of precision. You have to practice these skill sets so that you will not make a mistake and your opponent will not be able to use the same distracters on you for their advantage, I seen it.

Faking Maim

This is a method that is nothing new in the fight world, as well as real life. Everyone in their life time has lied, or fooled someone into getting results that they are looking for. Regardless of our religion or moral beliefs we all can say that lying is a part of life... It cannot be denied or defended. Now, how you tell that lie or how you perceived it to be, weather you get your results or not, it's still wrong, underhanded or just a flat out disservice in the sacrifice of honesty.

In this case I will use 52 Blocks Carolina Chaos style art of fighting and the term is called Faking Maim.

What is Faking Maim you wonder? Its only your own method of faking an injury to gain the advantage of your opponents offensive attack and strategic plans. In light, Faking that you are maimed It will be explained in small detail, but you won't have to be a rocket scientist to figure the rest out. So that it may fit into your arsenal, you must utilize your ability to have a good poker face and do what needs to be done to Fake and Maim.

You are in a scuffle and the fight is hot and heavy. The advantage seems to be going in his or her favor. Strategically allow yourself to enter his space and use trickery to make him think you've been injured by way of his hands or a mistake of your own. (Stink Face) should be automatic to display pain, discomfort and a loss of confidence so that your opponent may overload with an offensive barrage and allow him to make the mistake that is costly. This will make him think that you are hurt or maimed or out of commission. This sends off a brain stem spark and acknowledges that you are beat, or you have lost focus and can no longer defend yourself. But through this, your 52 Blocks should still be sharp, and your mind should be extremely focused on survival and a carefully planned out counter attack to turn the tides on the opponent and get yourself back in to the position to balance the fight or end the battle based on your ability to use Faking Maim to your advantage. Nothing is guaranteed because you are not the only fighter with skills, or the only fighter on the block with trickery skills. Know yourself and apply what you know to the situation at hand. It's up to you to do what you feel, but you have to do this in hopes it rears the best solution for what you are trying to accomplish. Prepare, and get what you need to win the battle or event at hand.

What Fuels Us

We have to look at what we eat and how we use that energy for training and conditioning. This section will give a bit more incite on what is good to eat, and what makes us as a warrior function. To be sure, what we eat can determine or output of energy and effectiveness of technique. What was said before, it's like putting 87 Grade gas in a 2017 Lamborghini Gallardo. It will not function properly, the car was made for a much higher grade of fuel, so that it will give you optimum performance. It goes the same with our body's, you have to treat it like a machine so that it could function at its best. Proper maintenance gives you superb and absolute results of working and performing at its best. Be aware of what is put into your body, it is a machine that requires maintence, and true attention to detail to make what you have work for you exactly when you need it.

Foods that are great eat range from so many different food groups. Learning these food groups will give you a better understand of what you want to put in your body. You will be responsible for the output that comes from your machine based on what is put into your mouth. Great foods, assist in provoking extraordinary results.

Salmon/Tuna	Cashews
Lean Chicken Breast	Peanuts
Steaks, Grass Fed are the best	Avocadoes
Whole Eggs	Lentils
Bison Burgers	Coconut Oils

These are some examples foods that are good for fighters, and people that want to improve their bodies to become well oiled machines. You are what you eat, and these foods are great for what you want to accomplished in changing your body to become so much more healthier.

Learning to eat in Moderation and getting exactly what is needed. Overeating is the quickest way to weight gain, even if it is healthy food.

Workout days should be consistent & go to a gym

Day 1 Chest, Arms, Calf

Day 2 Back, Traps, Shoulders, abs, Legs

Day 3 Chest, Arms, Calf's

Day 4 Back, Traps, Shoulders, Abs, Legs

Day 5 Cardio, Intense stretching,

Day 6 Rest

Day 7 Rest

Monitor and maintenance growth and performance. Speed, power, agility and endurance. With an emphasize on stamina. Mental preparedness is key to having a well balanced routine that creates gains and enhance performance. Consistent commitment is truly key to success and change of the body as well as mind. To see gains stay on track, if there are days where you cannot make it to the gym, replace with bodyweight exercises, pushups, pulls ups, squats, Dips, triceps dips.

These will keep the blood flowing till you get back to the gym. Remain active and you will remain ready.

Cardio is vital when it comes to building the perfect fighting machine. You have to remain consistent with your cardio, age does not matter although some seem to think. Running, jumping rope or even Machines will work just fine. But there is nothing as perfect as fight cardio, Though in my opinion is the best form of cardio needed to condition one's body to stay in fight shape and fight ready. The whole point of working your heart is to keep the body moving.

True purpose of cardio is the ability to go hard at a consistent level. It's not the fact of getting tired, it's all about being able to pace one's self and activate engine/heart and lungs to go as fast and as hard and still have the advantage if the fight goes as anticipated.

Conservation is key: But being in a mode of Controlled Chaos.... it can sometimes be no issue.

But allowing yourself a change to display an act of Controlled Chaos takes a very large amount of cardio, it can't be stressed enough. In order to be effective when it comes to fighting whether it be defensive or offensive, you have to be able to have the fuel to power through and remain vigilant. Extra cardio supplies focus, sharpness and most importantly.. Confidence.

Running at a consistent pace, sprints, Burpee's till it hurts. Jumping rope are great ways to improve your cardio. What will you do to increase your advantage, and make your body as lethal as possible. Again, there are many ways to do what you need to do for getting in shape. But how will you do it with a changed mind set and what it takes to maintain it. Get to work, don't stop, keep pushing till you are tired. Keep pushing till you can't go anymore. Are you throwing up yet?

The Just Of the Whole Movement

 Teaching basic boxing techniques and movements. All the blocks, parries, evades, takedowns strikes and conditioning drills. Explaining every technique and its uses. Present accurate history of 52 Blocks and the other names associated with it. Learn to give its origin, its top practitioners. Identify different ways of demonstrating their particular ways of implementing 52blocks. Explain ways each are different and how they are similar. Explain its effectiveness and why it's a valid and proven style of fighting. Explain and demonstrate its training regiment, workout routines, and why we do them. Having partners as I stated in earlier texts to help demonstrate is very important. The student of 52 blocks as to see and have hands on knowledge with the instructor, they need to see examples to show its true effectiveness. Presenting realness by throwing strikes full force is our method of staying tight and right. But we use extreme caution in all of our training exercises. It that is emphasized and stressed accordingly. The will always be pros and cons to each and every art. But that is reason why we practice our craft. With this we are able to prevail when our weaknesses are exposed. Never claiming to be a master or expert at 52 Block, but merely a practitioner of it as well as Innovator that has developed and effectiveness in that art. Using focus mitts for accuracy and sharpness and perfecting angle while striking. Use heavy bags for power and the development of torque. Jumping rope for agility of the feet and spring in knees. Extreme cardio is also developed from jumping rope, it's practically the best and most effective way to have raw cardio used to fight.

Body conditioning drills, shins, knees, thighs, stomach, Both side. Chest, upper back, shoulders, elbows, forearms, and complete hand. When conditioning the body, it is a slow but very consistent process. It takes time to harden shins, elbows, and hand. Preparing your mind is the first step, then the body will coordinate with the mind to become one whole conditioning and complete weapon. Preparation is the Key to maximize ones true potential. If you look back at all the great fighters in the world both past and present, you see that they had a workout routine to prepare and go into a fight with the best possible strategy possible. And it usually words out just fine based on how they prepared and what they prepared for. Easy planning is easy execution, easy execution means fluid and successful victory. Doing what is easy is one thing, but preparing and doing properly is another. Take the time to prepare, that is the best strategy.

What you call that?

Throughout the art of 52 Blocks, you find different practitioners having different names for their techniques. And there is nothing wrong with that. Every technique is presented differently and used alike in plenty of cases. They are designed to counter, block, attack or evade a certain skill set or a movement. With Carolina Chaos style of fighting, here are some techniques that are used in the art of 52 Blocks Carolina Chaos Style

Skull and Crossbones
Closed Door
Rob the Bank
Tyson
Achilles
Maze Runner

Ortho
Himalaya
Protect the Chest
Take it Back
Head Job
Complete Silence
Kryptonite
Sparta
L. Bogie
Art Of Running
Remove the Crown
Charlie's Horse
Push and Pop
Knuckle Up
Book Reader
Stutter Step
Butter Fly
Bum Rush
Spinning Back Fist
Peek-a-Boo
Take a Knee
Shoulder Brushes

Hand of God
Devil's Elbow
Getting Dirty
Straight Blast
Wrecking Ball
Rolling Hands
Broken Arrow
Blow Kisses
Catch and Kiss
Shoe Shine
Blue Reign
Dirty Hands
Ghetto Life
Make Em Limp
Busting Rocks
Shoulder Push
4 inches
Chin Check
Racking Ribs
Ring around the Collar
Breaking the Glass
Smashing

Shooters Regret
Shutter Down

There are many more that are used in the system, but these are the more prolific techniques used on a more consistent level.

Take your time; Repetition is the key to perfection. When teaching, I teach 3 things. Hit hard, Hit Fast, Hit first. It is very important to focus and know what techniques to execute and when to execute them.

Complete movements and allowing your body to adapt to what you are doing so that it will become second nature to you. With this, you will not have to think about what you are going to do, but you will simply know how to react to a situation when defending one's self or a third party. Always keep your hands and chest level, and moving. Never will you be in an offensive stance, or your hands clinched, they should always be open, relaxed and never tense. Let you punches flow, your feet glide, and chin tucked and ready to be an offensive threat or a defensive wizard.

52 Blocks is a culture, a community and a way of life. It will always be more than a fighting style, but never will it be a style of disruptive aptitude. Keep your ego in check, never allow your anger to take you away from the code of 52 Blocks which was stated by one of the foremost practitioners in 52 Blocks Diallo Fraizer

1. Freedom
2. Family
3. Liberation
4. Unity

Always practice your craft. Cardio is one of the most important key points within the art. In order to throw techniques at a fast and precise pace you have to be able to last when you train and when you fight. Keep your body up physically with training, keep your mind trained mentally with instruction and dedicate yourself to being great at whatever you do, not just in 52 Blocks, but in all endeavors of life. Stay safe.

Lemont D. Davis
Retired 3x World Kickboxing Champion
Retired MMA fighter
Black Belt in Various Marital Arts
52 Blocks Practitioner and Innovator.

Acknowledgements

Throughout my journey there have been pivotal people that have been a part of my life in the world of martial arts. They have been father figures, mentors, and friends. But first and foremost I'd like to thank God for the gift of creation. He blessed me with breath and an opportunity to become a powerful man of God, a Fantastic husband, and loving and fair father. I thank him for this ability that he has given me, no one else could do what he has done. I want to thank my wife for allowing me to train, and compete at such a consistent level. She has been my greatest support and critic. She is the best and I work hard and sacrifice a lot so that she may know that I do appreciate her. Love You Louise!!

I would like to Thank my Sensei John Ormsby and Bill McDonald. They gave me my start in the Marital Arts and saw great things in me and blessed me with their talents and wisdom of the martial arts. I thank them for everything they put in me, when I was hard headed, I paid for it. And when I was on point they let me know. But over all I feel they are truly proud of me and my accomplishments. I like to thank my Uncle Mac, he gave me an avenue to train with him in my early years, I give him all the credit to starting my career in the Martial Arts. Without him, I would not have been on the road to becoming a great Martial Artists. I am forever grateful for all that has been put upon my life. God has been good and he has never failed me. I'd like to thank Daniel Marks and the Solid brothers out of Constellation 52 Global out of Staten Island NY. They are the real pioneers and the most authentic instructors of the REAL 52 Blocks art form. If you want to learn the history, and the exact truth about 52 Blocks these guys are the proven warriors of the art. I appreciate their knowledge, brotherhood, and friendship. Last but not least my Grandma Essie, she gave up everything for me. She allowed me to go with John and Bill, she trusted them and they never let her down. She is a true angel, and a blessing to my life. She is a special woman with a lot of heart and compassion, and she is appreciated for taking me in when I was a year old. My mother left me on her door step and left me, and my Grandmother stepped up and took the responsibility of raising me into the great man that I am today. I am bless. I love you Grandma. And to all my true family, friends, opponents and fans out there. Thank you for your support both in the Kickboxing Ring, MMA Cage and in the Gym training and teaching. God Bless, and until the next book or training session. Be safe, Stay safe, so you won't have to be Defaced.

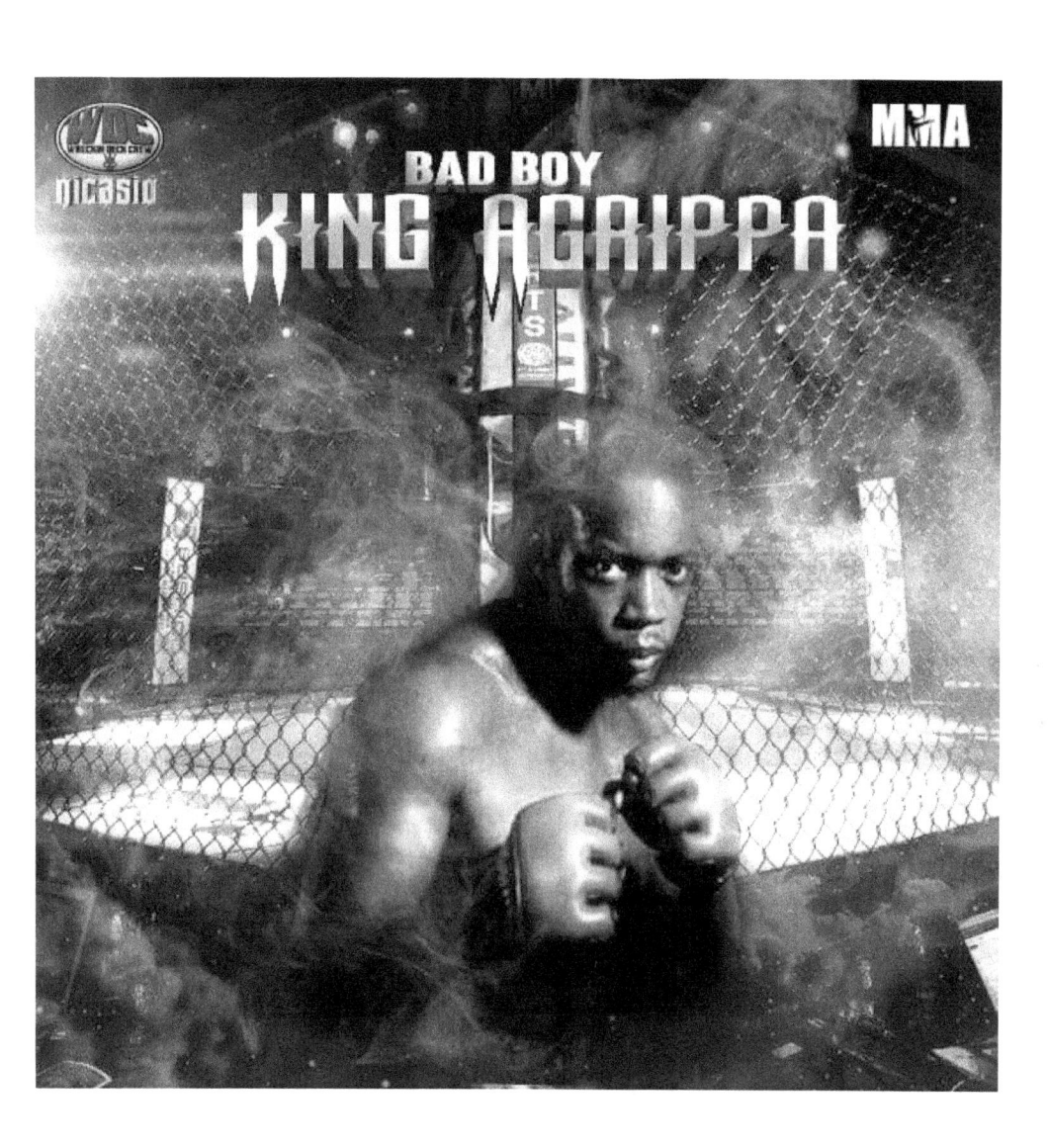

BAD BOY
KING AGRIPPA

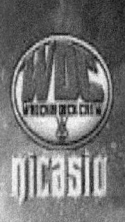

MMA

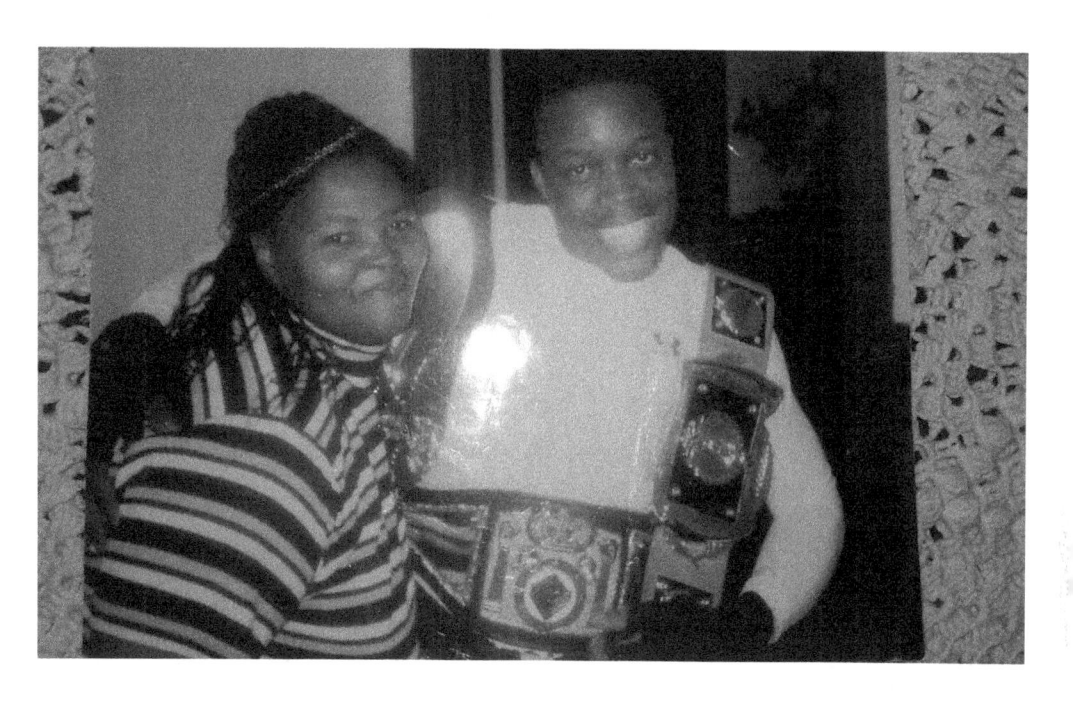

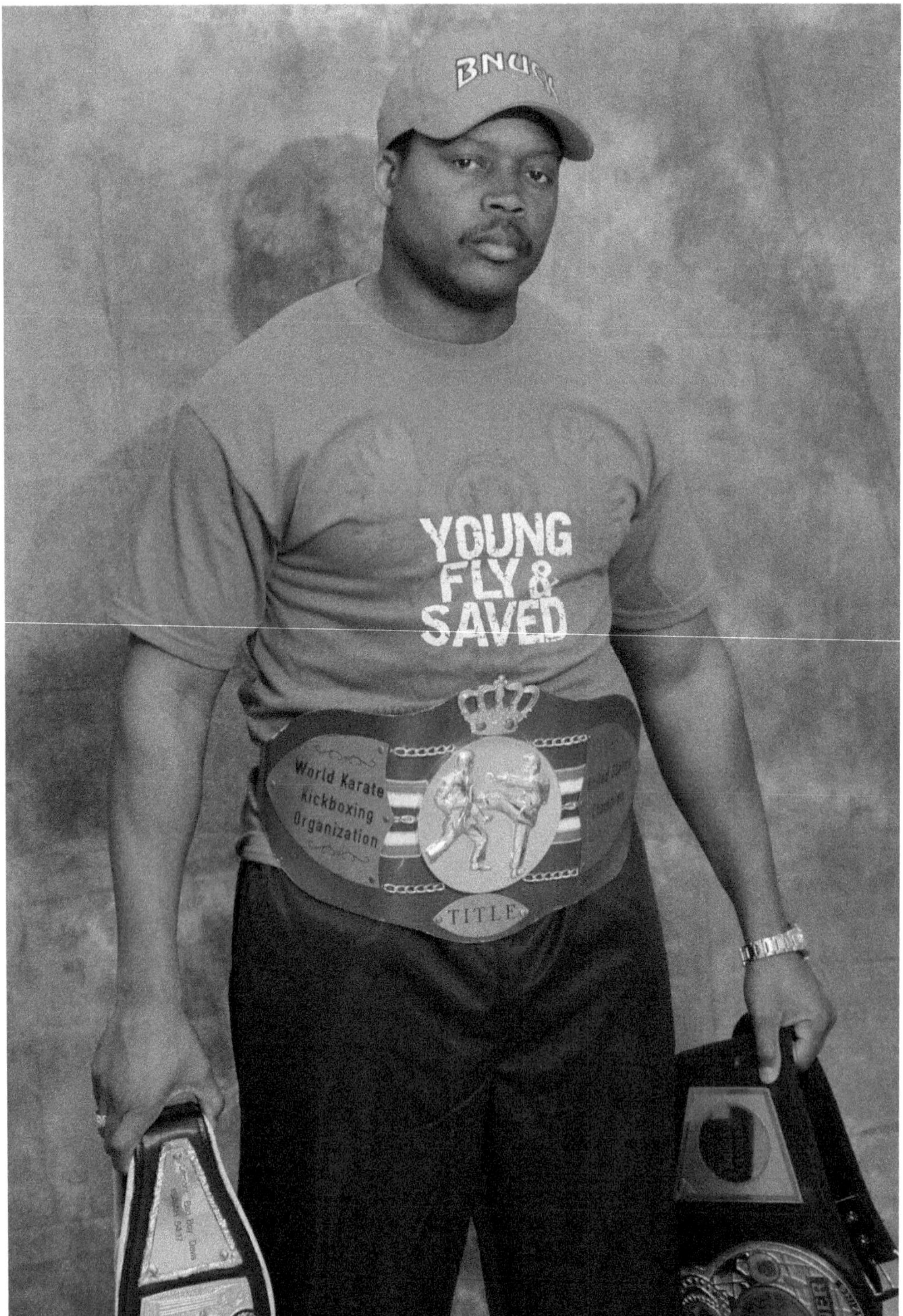
YOUNG
FLY &
SAVED
World Karate
Kickboxing
Organization
TITLE
WINNER